The Best Low Sodium Recipe Book

Boost Your Metabolism and Enjoy Your Meals with Incredibly Tasty Low Sodium Dishes

Jennifer Loyel

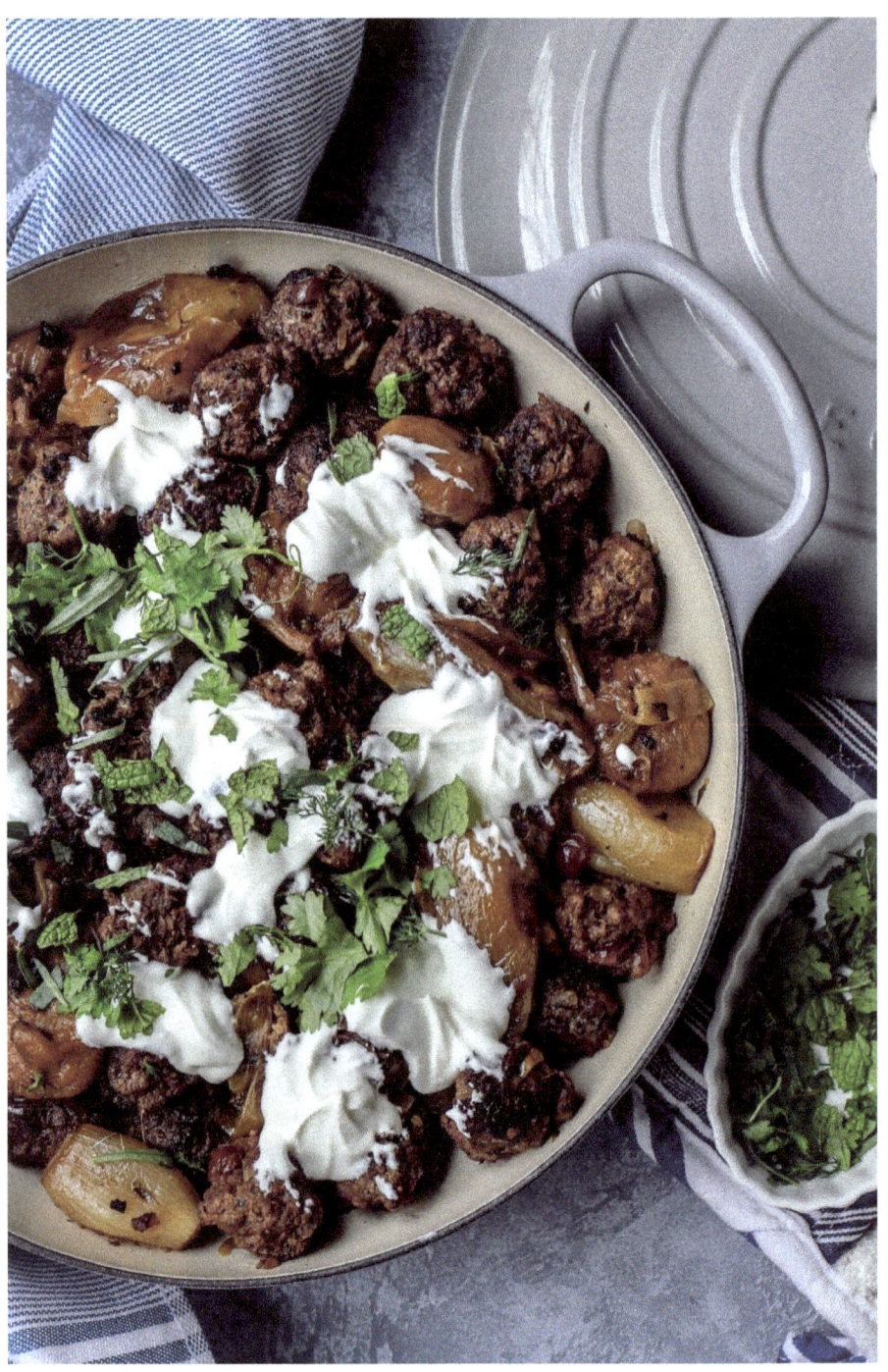

professional advice. The content within this book has been derived from various sources. Please consult a licensed professional before attempting any techniques outlined in this book.

By reading this document, the reader agrees that under no circumstances is the author responsible for any losses, direct or indirect, which are incurred as a result of the use of information contained within this document, including, but not limited to, — errors, omissions, or inaccuracies.

Table of Contents

Chicken With Pineapple Raisin Sauce

Servings: 4

Ingredients:

- 1 tablespoon olive oil
- 2 tablespoons unsalted butter
- 4 (6-ounce) boneless, skinless chicken breasts
- 3 tablespoons flour
- 1/2 teaspoon dried tarragon leaves
- 1/8 teaspoon pepper
- 1 medium onion, chopped
- 2 tablespoons minced fresh ginger root
- 2 (8-ounce) cans pineapple tidbits in juice
- 2 tablespoons lemon juice
- 2 tablespoons honey
- 1/3 cup golden raisins
- 1/3 cup raisins

Directions:

1. Melt olive oil and butter in large skillet over medium heat.
2. Meanwhile, sprinkle chicken with flour, tarragon, and pepper. Add to skillet and brown, about 3–4 minutes on each side,

turning once, until almost cooked. Remove from skillet.

3. Add onion and ginger root to skillet; cook, stirring to scrape up pan drippings, for 4–5 minutes until tender.

4. Add undrained pineapple, lemon juice, honey, golden raisins, and raisins and bring to a simmer. Simmer for 4–5 minutes.

5. Return chicken to skillet and cover with sauce. Cover skillet and simmer over low heat for 8–12 minutes or until chicken is cooked to 160°F.

Nutrition Info: (Per Serving):Calories: 370; Total Fat: 10 g; Saturated Fat: 4 g; Cholesterol: 80 mg; Protein: 28 g; Sodium: 79 mg; Potassium: 584 mg; Fiber: 1 g; Carbohydrates: 42 g; Sugar: 31 g

Southwestern Chicken Breasts

Servings: 4

Ingredients:

- 4 boneless skinless chicken breast halves
- 4 ounces (115 g) Swiss cheese
- For marinade:
- ⅓ cup (80 ml) vegetable oil
- ⅓ cup (80 ml) lime juice
- 2 tablespoons (18 g) green chiles, chopped
- ¼ teaspoon garlic powder

Directions:

1. In a 9-inch (23-cm) square glass baking pan stir together all of the marinade ingredients. Add chicken breasts and marinate, turning once, in the refrigerator, for at least 45 minutes. Remove the chicken from the marinade. Drain. Grill or sauté chicken over medium heat for 7 minutes. Turn. Continue cooking until done, 6 to 8 minutes longer. Top each chicken breast with a slice of cheese. Continue cooking until cheese begins to melt. Serve with salsa.

Nutrition Info: (Per Serving): 76 g water; 246 calories (70% from fat, 27% from protein, 4% from carb); 17 g protein; 19 g total fat; 3 g saturated fat; 5 g monounsaturated fat; 11 g polyunsaturated fat; 2 g carb; 0 g fiber; 0 g sugar; 11 mg calcium; 1 mg iron; 64 mg sodium; 210 mg potassium; 30 IU vitamin A; 8 mg vitamin C; 41 mg cholesterol

Chicken Shepherd's Pie

Servings: 6

Ingredients:

- 2 tablespoons (16 g) cornstarch
- 1 cup (235 ml) low sodium chicken broth
- 1 ½ cups (165 g) chicken, cooked and diced
- 12 ounces (340 g) frozen mixed vegetables
- 3 cups (675 g) mashed potatoes

Directions:

1. Mix the cornstarch with the broth. Heat until thickened and bubbly. Stir in chicken. Place in bottom of a 9 × 9-inch (23 × 23-cm) baking dish. Cook vegetables until almost tender. Spread over chicken mixture. Cover with prepared mashed potatoes. Heat under broiler until potatoes start to brown.

Nutrition Info: (Per Serving): 110 g water; 201 calories (12% from fat, 29% from protein, 59% from carb); 14 g protein; 3 g total fat; 1 g saturated fat; 1 g monounsaturated fat; 1 g polyunsaturated fat; 29 g carb; 4 g fiber; 3 g sugar; 29 mg calcium; 1 mg iron;

92 mg sodium; 475 mg potassium; 21 IU vitamin A; 22 mg vitamin C; 31 mg cholesterol

Roman Chicken

Servings: 4

Ingredients:

- 8 (6-ounce) boneless, skinless chicken thighs
- 2 tablespoons flour
- 1/4 teaspoon pepper
- 2 tablespoons olive oil
- 1 medium onion, chopped
- 4 cloves garlic, sliced
- 1 medium red bell pepper, chopped
- 3 tablespoons no-salt-added tomato paste
- 1 (14-ounce) can no-salt-added diced tomatoes, undrained
- 1/3 cup rosé or white wine
- 1/2 cup Chicken Stock
- 2 teaspoons fresh marjoram leaves
- 2 teaspoons fresh basil leaves
- 2 tablespoons lemon juice

Directions:

1. Sprinkle chicken with flour and pepper and set aside.

2. In large skillet, heat olive oil over medium heat. Add chicken and cook, turning once, until almost cooked through, about 7–9 minutes. Remove chicken from skillet and set aside.

3. Add onion and garlic to pan; cook and stir to remove pan drippings. Cook until tender, about 5 minutes. Add red bell pepper to pan; cook for 2 minutes longer.

4. Add tomato paste to skillet; cook for 2 minutes. Then add the undrained tomatoes, wine, and chicken stock and bring to a simmer.

5. Return chicken to pan and bring back to a simmer. Reduce heat to low, cover, and simmer for 20 minutes or until chicken is cooked to 165°F.

6. Stir in marjoram, basil, and lemon juice and serve immediately.

Nutrition Info: (Per Serving):Calories: 238; Total Fat: 10 g; Saturated Fat: 1 g; Cholesterol: 68 mg; Protein: 19 g; Sodium: 104 mg; Potassium: 641 mg; Fiber: 2 g; Carbohydrates: 13 g; Sugar: 5 g

Easy Slow-cooker Curry

Servings: 4

Ingredients:

- 1 onion, quartered
- 4 chicken thighs, skinned
- 2 cups (475 ml) no-salt-added stewed tomatoes
- 2 tablespoons (12.5 g) curry powder
- ¼ teaspoon garlic powder
- 6 ounces (170 g) no-salt-added frozen peas

Directions:

1. Place the onion in the bottom of the slow cooker. Layer the chicken on top. Combine the remaining ingredients and pour over. Cook on low for 8 to 10 hours or on high for 4 to 5 hours.

Nutrition Info: (Per Serving): 205 g water; 128 calories (16% from fat, 36% from protein, 49% from carb); 12 g protein; 2 g total fat; 1 g saturated fat; 1 g monounsaturated fat; 1 g polyunsaturated fat; 16 g carb; 5 g fiber; 7 g sugar; 72 mg calcium; 3 mg iron;

80 mg sodium; 508 mg potassium; 1109 IU vitamin A; 24 mg vitamin C; 34 mg cholesterol

Chicken Kabobs

Servings: 4

Ingredients:

- 18 ounces (504 g) pineapple chunks
- 1 teaspoon cumin
- 1 teaspoon coriander
- ⅛ teaspoon garlic powder
- 1 tablespoon (7.5 g) chili powder
- 1 teaspoon cilantro
- 2 tablespoons (30 g) plain low-fat yogurt
- 10 ounces (280 g) boneless skinless chicken breast
- 1 red bell pepper
- 1 onion
- 8 cherry tomatoes

Directions:

1. Drain pineapple, reserving juice. In a large bowl, Blend together spices and yogurt. Add juice from pineapple and stir to mix. Cut the chicken into cubes and add to the mixture. Cover and refrigerate for 1 to 1 ½ hours. Cut pepper and onion into cubes. Arrange chicken, pineapple, and vegetables on skewers. Grill

over medium heat about 10 minutes, turning and basting with remaining marinade frequently.

Nutrition Info: (Per Serving): 230 g water; 201 calories (15% from fat, 47% from protein, 38% from carb); 24 g protein; 3 g total fat; 1 g saturated fat; 1 g monounsaturated fat; 1 g polyunsaturated fat; 19 g carb; 3 g fiber; 13 g sugar; 67 mg calcium; 2 mg iron; 65 mg sodium; 613 mg potassium; 2031 IU vitamin A; 91 mg vitamin C; 61 mg cholesterol

Smoked Chicken

Servings: 8

Ingredients:

- ¼ teaspoon cayenne pepper
- ½ teaspoon black pepper
- 1 teaspoon brown sugar
- 1 large chicken, 4 to 6 pounds (1 ¾ to 2 ¾ kg)

Directions:

1. Combine the spices and rub into the chicken skin. Smoke for 6 to 8 hours, according to smoker instructions.

Nutrition Info: (Per Serving): 94 g water; 372 calories (47% from fat, 51% from protein, 2% from carb); 46 g protein; 19 g total fat; 5 g saturated fat; 8 g monounsaturated fat; 4 g polyunsaturated fat; 2 g carb; 0 g fiber; 2 g sugar; 24 mg calcium; 2 mg iron; 79 mg sodium; 415 mg potassium; 132 IU vitamin A; 0 mg vitamin C; 137 mg cholesterol

White Lasagna

Servings: 6

Ingredients:

- 8 ounces (225 g) lasagna noodles
- 1 cup (160 g) onion, sliced
- ½ cup (60 g) green bell pepper, sliced
- 3 tablespoons (45 g) unsalted butter
- 2 cups (220 g) cooked chicken, diced
- 2 cups (475 ml) skim milk
- ¼ cup (28 g) all-purpose flour
- ¼ teaspoon black pepper
- 2 teaspoons (10 ml) low sodium chicken bouillon
- 2 cups (220 g) Swiss cheese, shredded

Directions:

1. Cook the noodles until tender, drain, and set aside. In a large skillet, cook the onion and bell pepper in butter until tender. Stir in the chicken. Combine the remaining ingredients except the cheese. Add to skillet; cook and stir until thickened. In a well-greased baking dish, make alternate layers of noodles, chicken mixture, and cheese, starting with noodles

and ending with cheese. Bake, uncovered, for 30 minutes at 350°F (180°C, gas mark 4).

Nutrition Info: (Per Serving): 152 g water; 507 calories (40% from fat, 26% from protein, 34% from carb); 33 g protein; 22 g total fat; 13 g saturated fat; 6 g monounsaturated fat; 2 g polyunsaturated fat; 43 g carb; 2 g fiber; 2 g sugar; 489 mg calcium; 3 mg iron; 144 mg sodium; 422 mg potassium; 13 mg vitamin C; 92 mg cholesterol

Slow Cooker Chicken Risotto

Servings: 4

Ingredients:

- 2 tablespoons olive oil
- 2 (6-ounce) boneless, skinless chicken breasts, cut into cubes
- 1 medium onion, finely chopped
- 3 cloves garlic, minced
- 13/4 cups Arborio or other short-grain rice
- 42/3 cups Chicken Stock
- 1/2 pound asparagus
- 2 tablespoons minced chives
- 2 tablespoons unsalted butter
- 2 tablespoons grated Parmesan cheese

Directions:

1. In skillet, heat olive oil over medium-high heat. Add chicken breasts; cook until lightly browned on all sides, about 3–4 minutes. Remove to plate.

2. Add onion and garlic to skillet; cook and stir to remove pan drippings. Add rice to skillet; cook for 1 minute longer. Remove to 4-quart slow cooker.

3. Add chicken to slow cooker. Pour chicken stock over all and stir. Cover and cook on high for 2 hours or until rice is almost tender; stir.

4. Rinse asparagus and slice into 1" pieces; add to slow cooker and stir. Cover and cook on high for another 25–35 minutes or until rice is tender, chicken is 160°F, and asparagus is tender.

5. Stir in chives, butter, and cheese; let stand 5 minutes, then serve.

Nutrition Info: (Per Serving):Calories: 517; Total Fat: 16 g; Saturated Fat: 6 g; Cholesterol: 51 mg; Protein: 26 g; Sodium: 140 mg; Potassium: 583 mg; Fiber: 1 g; Carbohydrates: 65 g; Sugar: 1 g

Broth-injected Turkey

Servings: 24

Ingredients:

- 12 pound (5 kg) turkey
- 1 cup (235 ml) low sodium chicken broth or turkey broth

Directions:

1. Preheat the oven to 500°F (250°C, gas mark 10). Using a hypodermic needle or baster-injector, inject the broth into the turkey. Let cook for 20 minutes or until the exterior is crisp, but not golden brown. Reduce heat to 375°F (190°C, gas mark 5). Let turkey roast until finished.

Nutrition Info: (Per Serving): 112 g water; 177 calories (22% from fat, 78% from protein, 0% from carb); 33 g protein; 4 g total fat; 1 g saturated fat; 1 g monounsaturated fat; 1 g polyunsaturated fat; 0 g carb; 0 g fiber; 0 g sugar; 21 mg calcium; 2 mg iron; 110 mg sodium; 457 mg potassium; 0 IU vitamin A; 0 mg vitamin C; 103 mg cholesterol

Pasta With Chicken And Vegetables

Servings: 6

Ingredients:

- 8 ounces (230 g) linguine or spaghetti
- 2 tablespoons (30 ml) vegetable oil
- 2 small zucchini, cut into strips
- ½ cup (35 g) mushrooms, sliced
- 1 clove garlic, minced
- ½ teaspoon dried basil
- 1 cup (235 ml) skim milk
- 2 cups (220 g) chicken, cooked and cubed
- ⅛ teaspoon black pepper
- 6 roma tomatoes, sliced
- 2 tablespoons (10 g) Parmesan cheese, grated

Directions:

1. Cook linguine or spaghetti according to package directions. In a skillet, Heat the oil. Add the zucchini, mushrooms, garlic, and basil. Cook and stir until zucchini is crisp-tender, 2 to 3 minutes. Drain pasta and return to pan. Stir in milk, chicken, pepper, and

zucchini mixture and heat through. Add tomatoes and cheese. Toss and serve.

Nutrition Info: (Per Serving): 76 g water; 301 calories (31% from fat, 29% from protein, 40% from carb); 21 g protein; 10 g total fat; 2 g saturated fat; 3 g monounsaturated fat; 4 g polyunsaturated fat; 30 g carb; 1 g fiber; 0 g sugar; 103 mg calcium; 1 mg iron; 104 mg sodium; 302 mg potassium; 146 IU vitamin A; 1 mg vitamin C; 80 mg cholesterol

Apple Chicken

Servings: 4

Ingredients:

- 4 (6-ounce) boneless, skinless chicken breasts
- 1/4 cup flour
- 1/2 teaspoon dried thyme leaves
- 1/8 teaspoon white pepper
- 2 tablespoons unsalted butter
- 1 tablespoon olive oil
- 2 unpeeled Granny Smith apples, thickly sliced
- 11/2 cups apple juice
- 2 tablespoons lemon juice
- 3 tablespoons Honey Mustard
- 3 tablespoons sliced green onions
- 1/2 cup chopped toasted pecans

Directions:

1. Sprinkle chicken breasts with flour, thyme, and pepper.
2. In large skillet, heat butter and olive oil over medium heat until melted. Add chicken; cook,

turning once, until golden brown, about 5–7
minutes. Remove chicken from skillet.

3.   To drippings remaining in skillet, add apples;
sauté for 2 minutes. Add apple juice, lemon
juice, and honey mustard to skillet and bring
to a simmer.

4.   Return chicken to skillet; reduce heat to low
and simmer for another 7–9 minutes or until
chicken is thoroughly cooked to 160°F.
Sprinkle with green onions and toasted pecans
and serve.

Nutrition Info: (Per Serving):Calories: 739; Total Fat:
37 g; Saturated Fat: 7 g; Cholesterol: 161 mg; Protein:
60 g; Sodium: 125 mg; Potassium: 779 mg; Fiber: 6 g;
Carbohydrates: 42 g; Sugar: 25 g

Turkey And Zucchini Meatloaf

Servings: 8

Ingredients:

- 1 ¼ pounds (570 g) ground turkey
- 1 cup zucchini, grated
- ½ cup (60 g) low sodium bread crumbs
- 1 egg
- 1 tablespoon (0.4 g) dried parsley
- ½ teaspoon black pepper
- ½ teaspoon garlic powder
- 1 teaspoon onion powder
- ¼ cup (80 g) peach preserves
- 2 teaspoons (10 g) Dijon mustard

Directions:

1. Preheat oven to 350°F (180°C, gas mark 4). Combine first 8 ingredients In a large bowl and mix well. Shape mixture into a loaf on a baking sheet. Bake for 45 minutes. Stir the preserves and the mustard together. Spread on top of the loaf. Return to oven until internal temperature is 165°F, about 20 minutes.

Nutrition Info: (Per Serving): 71 g water; 191 calories (23% from fat, 49% from protein, 28% from carb); 23

g protein; 5 g total fat; 1 g saturated fat; 1 g monounsaturated fat; 1 g polyunsaturated fat; 13 g carb; 1 g fiber; 6 g sugar; 42 mg calcium; 2 mg iron; 68 mg sodium; 293 mg potassium; 108 IU vitamin A; 4 mg vitamin C; 85 mg cholesterol

Chicken Cacciatore

Servings: 4

Ingredients:

- 4 teaspoons olive oil
- 1 large sweet onion, diced or sliced
- 4 (4-ounce) boneless, skinless chicken breasts
- 1/4 teaspoon freshly ground black pepper
- 2 tablespoons dry red wine
- 1 (15-ounce) can no-salt-added tomato sauce
- 1 teaspoon garlic powder
- 1/2 teaspoon dried basil
- 1/4 teaspoon dried oregano
- 1/4 teaspoon dried parsley
- 1/8 teaspoon mustard powder
- Pinch grated lemon zest
- Pinch dried red pepper flakes
- 1 teaspoon lemon juice
- 1/4 teaspoon granulated sugar
- Optional: 4 tablespoons grated Parmesan cheese

Directions:

1. Heat a deep nonstick skillet over medium heat. Add the olive oil and chopped onion; sauté the onion until transparent. Push to the edges of the pan.

2. Add the chicken breasts. Sprinkle the pepper over the chicken. Pan-fry for 2 minutes on each side. Use tongs to transfer the chicken breasts to a bowl or platter; set aside.

3. Add the wine to the pan. Bring to a boil and cook for 2 minutes, stirring the wine into the onion and using a spoon or spatula to scrape (deglaze) the bottom of the pan.

4. Add the tomato sauce, garlic powder, basil, oregano, parsley, mustard powder, lemon zest, red pepper flakes, lemon juice, and sugar to the pan; stir to combine.

5. Add the chicken back to the pan, spooning some of the tomato sauce over the top of the chicken. Reduce heat. Simmer, covered, for 25–35 minutes or until chicken is cooked to 160°F. Serve immediately, topped with freshly grated Parmesan cheese if desired.

Nutrition Info: (Per Serving):Calories: 247; Total Fat: 6 g; Saturated Fat: 1 g; Cholesterol: 65 mg; Protein: 28 g; Sodium: 92 mg; Potassium: 799 mg; Fiber: 2 g; Carbohydrates: 16 g; Sugar: 10 g

Chicken-broccoli Pie

Servings: 6

Ingredients:

- 1 cup (110 g) cooked chicken, cubed
- 1 cup (70 g) broccoli, chopped
- 1 cup (180 g) tomatoes, chopped
- 1 cup (160 g) onion, chopped
- ¼ cup (25 g) Parmesan cheese, grated
- 1 cup (235 ml) skim milk
- ½ cup (55 g) Buttermilk Baking Mix
- 2 eggs
- ¼ teaspoon black pepper

Directions:

1. Heat oven to 400°F (200°C, gas mark 6) and grease a 9-inch (23-cm) pie plate. Mix chicken, veggies, and cheese and spoon evenly into pie plate. Beat milk, baking mix, eggs, and pepper in the blender or with a wire whisk until smooth. Pour evenly over the chicken mixture. Bake for about 35 minutes, or until a knife inserted in the center comes out clean. Let stand for 5 minutes before cutting.

Nutrition Info: (Per Serving): 144 g water; 163 calories (33% from fat, 33% from protein, 34% from carb); 13 g protein; 6 g total fat; 2 g saturated fat; 2 g monounsaturated fat; 1 g polyunsaturated fat; 14 g carb; 2 g fiber; 3 g sugar; 149 mg calcium; 1 mg iron; 132 mg sodium; 315 mg potassium; 759 IU vitamin A; 18 mg vitamin C; 103 mg cholesterol

Chicken And Dumplings

Servings: 6

Ingredients:

- 1 ½ cups (165 g) chicken, cooked and cubed
- 3 cups (705 ml) low sodium chicken broth
- 3 cups (705 ml) water
- 1 ½ cups (195 g) carrot, sliced
- 4 medium potatoes, peeled and cubed
- 1 onion, chopped
- For dumplings:
- 2 cups (220 g) all-purpose flour
- 1 tablespoon (14 g) sodium-free baking powder
- 6 tablespoons (85 g) unsalted butter
- ⅔ cup (157 ml) skim milk

Directions:

1. Place chicken, broth, water, and vegetables In a large pan. Bring to boiling. To make the dumplings, stir together the dry ingredients. Cut in butter until mixture resembles coarse crumbs. Stir in liquid until dough holds together in a ball. Drop dumplings on top by

tablespoonfuls. Reduce heat and simmer uncovered for 10 minutes. Cover and simmer for 10 minutes more.

Nutrition Info: (Per Serving): 489 g water; 546 calories (25% from fat, 16% from protein, 59% from carb); 22 g protein; 16 g total fat; 8 g saturated fat; 4 g monounsaturated fat; 1 g polyunsaturated fat; 81 g carb; 6 g fiber; 4 g sugar; 200 mg calcium; 4 mg iron; 122 mg sodium; 1325 mg potassium; 4287 IU vitamin A; 18 mg vitamin C; 62 mg cholesterol

Chicken Liver Stroganoff

Servings: 4

Ingredients:

- 1 cup (160 g) onion, chopped
- 2 tablespoons (28 g) unsalted butter
- ½ pound (225 g) chicken livers
- 8 ounces (225 g) mushrooms, sliced
- 1 tablespoon (7 g) paprika
- 1 cup (230 g) sour cream

Directions:

1. Cook onion in butter until just tender. Add livers and mushrooms. Stir in paprika. Cover and cook over low heat until livers are done, about 10 minutes. Stir in sour cream and cook until just heated. Serve over rice or noodles.

Nutrition Info: (Per Serving): 151 g water; 262 calories (68% from fat, 18% from protein, 14% from carb); 12 g protein; 20 g total fat; 12 g saturated fat; 5 g monounsaturated fat; 1 g polyunsaturated fat; 10 g carb; 2 g fiber; 3 g sugar; 85 mg calcium; 5 mg iron; 60 mg sodium; 445 mg potassium; 15 mg vitamin C; 221 mg cholesterol

Fried Chicken

Servings: 8

Ingredients:

- 1 chicken, cut into pieces, 3 to 4 pounds (1 ½ to 1 ¾ kg)
- For marinade:
- 2 cups (475 ml) buttermilk
- ¼ cup (60 g) Dijon mustard
- 1 tablespoon (9 g) onion powder
- 1 teaspoon dry mustard
- 1 teaspoon cayenne pepper
- 1 teaspoon black pepper
- For coating:
- 3 cups (330 g) all-purpose flour
- 1 tablespoon (14 g) sodium-free baking powder
- 1 tablespoon (9 g) garlic powder
- 1 tablespoon (9 g) onion powder
- 1 tablespoon (9 g) dry mustard
- 1 tablespoon cayenne pepper
- 1 ½ teaspoons black pepper

Directions:

1. Cut chicken into pieces. In a 1-gallon resealable plastic bag, Combine marinade ingredients. Add chicken pieces. Seal bag and turn to coat chicken evenly. Refrigerate at least overnight and up to 2 days, turning occasionally. Whisk together coating ingredients in a 9 × 13-inch (23 × 33-cm) baking dish. Add chicken pieces to dish, allowing as much marinade to stay on the chicken as you can. Turn to coat evenly and thickly. Let stand in coating mix 1 to 2 hours, turning occasionally. Chicken will continue to absorb flour. The idea is to get a thick coating completely covering the chicken to seal in the juices when it's fried. Heat oil to a depth of at least 1 ½ inches (4 cm) in a deep fryer or heavy frying pan. Heat to 350°F (180°C, gas mark 4). Add 4 pieces of chicken. Reduce heat to 300°F (150°C, gas mark 2). Fry for 5 minutes. Turn carefully to avoid breaking coating. Fry until done through, about 15 minutes depending on size of pieces. Reheat oil to 350°F (180°C, gas mark 4) and fry the

remaining 4 pieces the same way. Serve hot or cold.

Nutrition Info: (Per Serving): 88 g water; 247 calories (8% from fat, 21% from protein, 70% from carb); 13 g protein; 2 g total fat; 1 g saturated fat; 1 g monounsaturated fat; 1 g polyunsaturated fat; 43 g carb; 2 g fiber; 4 g sugar; 182 mg calcium; 3 mg iron; 91 mg sodium; 458 mg potassium; 412 IU vitamin A; 3 mg vitamin C; 20 mg cholesterol

Grilled Jerk Chicken

Servings: 4

Ingredients:

- 1 teaspoon Jerk Spice Blend
- 1 teaspoon Bragg Liquid Aminos
- 2 teaspoons fresh lime juice
- 1 teaspoon olive or canola oil
- 1 jalapeño, seeded and chopped
- 2 scallions, white and green parts chopped
- 1 teaspoon granulated sugar
- Pinch mustard powder
- 4 (4-ounce) boneless, skinless chicken breasts

Directions:

1. Preheat a George Foreman–style indoor grill.
2. Add all ingredients except the chicken to a small food processor or blender and purée.
3. Rub both sides of the chicken with the spice mixture. Grill for 4–6 minutes, until the chicken is cooked through to 160°F. Serve immediately.

Nutrition Info: (Per Serving):Calories: 141; Total Fat: 2 g; Saturated Fat: 0 g; Cholesterol: 65 mg; Protein:

26 g; Sodium: 133 mg; Potassium: 315 mg; Fiber: 0 g; Carbohydrates: 1 g; Sugar: 1 g

Chicken Pot Pie

Servings: 8

Ingredients:

- 1 chicken
- 2 cups (475 ml) low sodium chicken broth
- 1 onion, coarsely chopped
- 2 cups (260 g) carrot, sliced
- 6 ounces (170 g) no-salt-added frozen peas
- 1 tablespoon (0.4 g) dried parsley
- 1 teaspoon dried thyme
- ⅔ cup (73 g) all-purpose flour
- 1 cup (235 ml) water
- 6 cups (1350 g) mashed potatoes

Directions:

1. Place chicken and broth in a slow cooker or Dutch oven and cook until chicken is done. Remove chicken from broth, debone, and chop coarsely. Strain fat from broth and add enough water to make 5 cups (1175 ml). Return broth to ovenproof Dutch oven. Add onion, carrot, peas, and spices and cook until carrots are tender. Add flour to water in a jar

46

with a tight-fitting lid. Shake until dissolved. Add to broth and cook until thickened. Stir in chicken. Prepare mashed potatoes and drop onto top of chicken mixture. Place under broiler until potatoes start to brown.

Nutrition Info: (Per Serving): 111 g water; 231 calories (4% from fat, 19% from protein, 77% from carb); 11 g protein; 1 g total fat; 0 g saturated fat; 0 g monounsaturated fat; 0 g polyunsaturated fat; 45 g carb; 5 g fiber; 4 g sugar; 36 mg calcium; 2 mg iron; 96 mg sodium; 609 mg potassium; 4360 IU vitamin A; 36 mg vitamin C; 17 mg cholesterol

Tandoori Chicken

Servings: 8

Ingredients:

- 1 cup (230 g) plain low-fat yogurt
- ½ teaspoon cardamom
- ½ teaspoon cumin
- ½ teaspoon turmeric
- ⅛ teaspoon cayenne pepper
- 1 teaspoon bay leaf, crushed
- ½ teaspoon garlic powder
- ¾ teaspoon ground ginger
- ¼ cup (40 g) minced onion
- ¼ cup (60 ml) lime juice
- ¼ teaspoon black pepper
- 1 teaspoon ground cinnamon
- 1 teaspoon coriander
- 8 chicken thighs

Directions:

1. Combine yogurt with all other spices, mixing well. Prick chicken with a fork. In a plastic food bag or glass pan large enough to hold the chicken, cover the chicken with yogurt marinade, making sure all surfaces of the

chicken are coated. Cover and refrigerate for a minimum of 3 hours, but overnight is best. Turn at least once while marinating. Grill over medium coals until done or place chicken in a greased roasting pan with marinade and cook at 375°F (190°C, gas mark 5) for 45 minutes to 1 hour or until chicken is tender.

Nutrition Info: (Per Serving): 64 g water; 82 calories (24% from fat, 49% from protein, 28% from carb); 10 g protein; 2 g total fat; 1 g saturated fat; 1 g monounsaturated fat; 0 g polyunsaturated fat; 6 g carb; 1 g fiber; 3 g sugar; 75 mg calcium; 1 mg iron; 58 mg sodium; 232 mg potassium; 70 IU vitamin A; 5 mg vitamin C; 36 mg cholesterol

Honey Chicken

Servings: 4

Ingredients:

- 2 ½ tablespoons (35 ml) vegetable oil, divided
- 1 pound (455 g) sliced boneless chicken breast
- 1 egg
- ⅓ cup (43 g) cornstarch
- 2 onions, sliced
- 1 green bell pepper, sliced
- 6 ounces (170 g) snow peas
- ¼ cup (85 g) honey
- 2 tablespoons (16 g) sliced almonds

Directions:

1. Heat 1 ½ (25 ml) tablespoons of the oil in a wok. Dip half the chicken in the egg and dust with cornstarch. Stir-fry until just cooked, 4 to 5 minutes. Remove and repeat with remaining chicken. Remove; add the rest of the oil to the wok. Stir-fry the onion until it begins to soften. Add the pepper and snow peas and stir-fry until crisp cooked, about 4 minutes.

Add the honey and toss the vegetables in it until well coated. Add the chicken and toss until coated and heated through. Sprinkle the almonds over the top.

Nutrition Info: (Per Serving): 216 g water; 466 calories (32% from fat, 34% from protein, 34% from carb); 40 g protein; 17 g total fat; 3 g saturated fat; 6 g monounsaturated fat; 7 g polyunsaturated fat; 39 g carb; 3 g fiber; 23 g sugar; 71 mg calcium; 3 mg iron 112 mg sodium; 590 mg potassium; 695 IU vitamin A; 59 mg vitamin C; 158 mg cholesterol

Quick Indoor-grilled Chicken Breast

Servings: 4

Ingredients:

- 4 (4-ounce) boneless, skinless chicken breasts
- 1 teaspoon frozen apple juice concentrate
- 4 tablespoons sodium-free honey mustard sauce
- 1 teaspoon lemon juice
- 1 teaspoon Citrus Pepper

Directions:

1. Plug in indoor grill. Add chicken. Close the lid. Grill for 4–6 minutes or until the chicken is cooked to 160°F.
2. While the chicken grills, add the remaining ingredients to a small microwave-safe bowl. Immediately before serving, microwave on high for 30 seconds to heat the sauce. Evenly divide over the grilled chicken breasts and serve immediately.

Nutrition Info: (Per Serving):Calories: 141; Total Fat: 1 g; Saturated Fat: 0 g; Cholesterol: 65 mg; Protein:

26 g; Sodium: 74 mg; Potassium: 312 mg; Fiber: 0 g; Carbohydrates: 2 g; Sugar: 1 g

Chicken Paella

Servings: 6

Ingredients:

- 1 ¼ pounds (570 g) boneless chicken breast, cut into strips
- 1 tablespoon (15 ml) olive oil
- 1 onion, chopped
- 2 cloves garlic, minced
- 2 ¼ cups (535 ml) low sodium chicken broth
- 1 cup (185 g) long-grain rice, uncooked
- 1 teaspoon dried oregano, crushed
- ½ teaspoon paprika
- ¼ teaspoon black pepper
- ⅛ teaspoon ground turmeric
- 2 cups (475 ml) low sodium stewed tomatoes, cut up
- 1 medium red bell pepper, cut into strips
- ¾ cup (98 g) frozen peas

Directions:

1. Rinse chicken; pat dry with paper towels. In a 10-inch (25-cm) skillet, cook chicken, half at a time, in hot oil until no longer pink. Remove

chicken from skillet. Add onion and garlic to skillet; cook until tender but not brown. Remove skillet from heat. Add broth, uncooked rice, oregano, paprika, black pepper, and turmeric. Bring to boiling. Reduce heat. Simmer covered for about 15 minutes. Add undrained tomatoes, bell pepper, and frozen peas to skillet. Cover and simmer about 5 minutes more or until rice is tender. Stir in cooked chicken. Cook and stir about 1 minute more or until heated through.

Nutrition Info: (Per Serving): 294 g water; 291 calories (12% from fat, 38% from protein, 49% from carb); 28 g protein; 4 g total fat; 1 g saturated fat; 2 g monounsaturated fat; 1 g polyunsaturated fat; 36 g carb; 3 g fiber; 5 g sugar; 66 mg calcium; 3 mg iron; 122 mg sodium; 652 mg potassium; 1434 IU vitamin A; 64 mg vitamin C; 55 mg cholesterol

Curried Black Bean And Turkey Salad

Servings: 8

Ingredients:

- ¾ cup (188 g) dried black beans
- ¾ cup (188 g) dried black-eyed peas
- 1 onion, chopped
- 2 cups (220 g) smoked turkey, chopped
- 1 cup (235 ml) Italian Dressing
- ¼ cup (15 g) fresh cilantro, chopped
- 2 teaspoons (4 g) curry powder
- ½ teaspoon red pepper flakes
- 1 cup (160 g) green onions, chopped
- 1 ⅓ cups (170 g) red bell pepper, chopped
- 1 ¼ cups (163 g) frozen corn, thawed

Directions:

1. Place dried beans and peas in separate saucepans. Cover with water. Add half of onion to each. Bring to a boil and boil 1 minute. Remove from heat, cover, and let stand for 1 hour. Add additional water to saucepans if needed. Divide turkey between pans. Simmer 1 hour or until tender. Drain. Combine beans, peas, and turkey In a large

bowl. Combine Italian dressing, cilantro, curry powder and, red pepper flakes. Pour over turkey and bean mixture while hot. Add green onion, pepper, and corn. Toss to mix. Cover and refrigerate overnight.

Nutrition Info: (Per Serving): 109 g water; 253 calories (35% from fat, 25% from protein, 40% from carb); 16 g protein; 10 g total fat; 2 g saturated fat; 2 g monounsaturated fat; 4 g polyunsaturated fat; 26 g carb; 5 g fiber; 6 g sugar; 66 mg calcium; 2 mg iron; 88 mg sodium; 603 mg potassium; 715 IU vitamin A; 29 mg vitamin C; 24 mg cholesterol

Blackened Chicken

Servings: 4

Ingredients:

- 4 chicken thighs
- 2 tablespoons (28 g) unsalted butter, melted
- 5 teaspoons (12.5 g) Cajun Blackening Spice Mix

Directions:

1. Trim excess fat from the chicken. Cut slashes through the skin and ½ inch (1 ¼ cm) deep to allow spices to penetrate the meat. Brush the thighs with the melted butter, then rub the spices in. Cook on a medium grill for about 25 minutes.

Nutrition Info: (Per Serving): 32 g water; 100 calories (67% from fat, 33% from protein, 0% from carb); 8 g protein; 7 g total fat; 4 g saturated fat; 2 g monounsaturated fat; 1 g polyunsaturated fat; 0 g carb; 0 g fiber; 0 g sugar; 6 mg calcium; 0 mg iron; 36 mg sodium; 96 mg potassium; 204 IU vitamin A; 0 mg vitamin C; 49 mg cholesterol

Steamed Chili-peppered Chicken

Servings: 4

Ingredients:

- 1/4 teaspoon ground ancho pepper
- 1/4 teaspoon ground chipotle pepper
- 1/8 teaspoon dried marjoram
- Pinch ground cumin
- 1/4 teaspoon dried Mexican oregano
- 1/8 teaspoon dried thyme
- 1/8 teaspoon ground cloves
- 1 teaspoon garlic powder
- 1 tablespoon white wine vinegar
- 4 (4-ounce) boneless, skinless chicken thighs

Directions:

1. In a small bowl, mix together the ancho pepper, chipotle pepper, marjoram, cumin, oregano, thyme, cloves, and garlic powder.
2. In a separate bowl, pour the vinegar over the chicken, turning the chicken to evenly coat it in the vinegar.
3. Cut out four 16" squares of parchment paper. Dip the vinegar-coated chicken in the

seasoning mixture, coating both sides. Place each thigh in the center of a parchment-paper square. Bring the 4 corners together and tie closed with string. Place in a steamer and steam over simmering water for 1 hour or until chicken is cooked to 160°F.

Nutrition Info: (Per Serving):Calories: 52; Total Fat: 1 g; Saturated Fat: 0 g; Cholesterol: 34 mg; Protein: 8 g; Sodium: 38 mg; Potassium: 108 mg; Fiber: 0 g; Carbohydrates: 0 g; Sugar: 0 g

Barbecued Chicken Sandwiches

Servings: 6

Ingredients:

- 2 cups (220 g) smoked chicken, shredded
- For sauce:
- 8 ounces (230 g) no-salt-added tomato sauce
- ¼ cup (60 ml) vinegar
- ¼ cup (85 g) molasses
- ½ teaspoon onion powder
- ½ teaspoon chili powder
- ½ teaspoon dry mustard
- ¼ teaspoon cayenne pepper
- ¼ teaspoon garlic powder

Directions:

1. Mix together sauce ingredients. Combine with chicken or spoon over chicken on the roll as desired.

Nutrition Info: (Per Serving): 76 g water; 147 calories (22% from fat, 39% from protein, 39% from carb); 14 g protein; 4 g total fat; 1 g saturated fat; 1 g monounsaturated fat; 1 g polyunsaturated fat; 14 g carb; 1 g fiber; 10 g sugar; 43 mg calcium; 2 mg iron;

50 mg sodium; 479 mg potassium; 249 IU vitamin A; 5 mg vitamin C; 42 mg cholesterol

Chicken Gyros

Servings: 4

Ingredients:

- 2 boneless chicken breasts, cut into 1/2-inch (1 1/4-cm) strips
- 2 tablespoons (30 g) low sodium ketchup
- 2 tablespoons (30 ml) olive oil
- 1 ½ teaspoons white wine vinegar
- 1 teaspoon dried oregano
- 1 teaspoon dry mustard
- 1 ½ teaspoons curry powder
- 4 pita breads, cut in half
- 1 ½ cups (30 g) lettuce, shredded
- ½ cup (90 g) tomato, chopped
- 1 cup (230 g) plain low-fat yogurt

Directions:

1. Place the chicken strips side by side in a glass baking dish. Stir together the ketchup, olive oil, white wine vinegar, oregano, mustard, and curry powder. Pour over the chicken in the dish. Allow the chicken to marinate while you Preheat the oven's broiler. Broil uncovered for 15 minutes with the meat

about 6 inches (15 cm) from the heat. Cook just until the chicken is cooked through, but not browned. Place hot chicken into pita pockets and spoon some of the juices from the pan over it. Top with lettuce, tomato, and yogurt.

Nutrition Info: (Per Serving): 133 g water; 325 calories (27% from fat, 21% from protein, 52% from carb); 17 g protein; 10 g total fat; 2 g saturated fat; 6 g monounsaturated fat; 42 g carb; 2 g Fiber;184 mg calcium; 3 mg iron; 93 mg sodium; 415 mg potassium; 341 IU vitamin A; 6 mg vitamin C; 26 mg cholesterol

Poached Chicken Breasts

Servings: 6–8

Ingredients:

- 8 (6-ounce boneless or 10-ounce bone-in) chicken breast halves
- 1 bay leaf
- 1/2 teaspoon black peppercorns
- 1 teaspoon mustard seeds
- 2 sprigs marjoram
- 1 square cheesecloth

Directions:

1. Place chicken in a large pot or saucepan. Place bay leaf, peppercorns, mustard seeds, and marjoram on a square of cheesecloth and tie with kitchen string; add to pot with chicken.
2. Cover everything in the pot with water. Bring to a simmer over medium heat, then reduce heat to medium-low. No bubbles should form in the center of the pot.
3. Cook the bone-in, skin-on chicken breasts for 18–22 minutes; cook boneless, skinless

chicken breasts for 12–15 minutes until 160°F.

4.   Remove pan from heat; remove chicken from pan and place in glass baking dish. Remove and discard the cheesecloth bundle. Pour some of the poaching liquid over the chicken; reserve the rest for another use.

5.   Cover the pan and refrigerate the chicken until cold. Remove bones and skin, if using bone-in breasts, and cube the meat. You can freeze the meat up to 4 months; to thaw, let stand overnight in the refrigerator.

Nutrition Info: (Per Serving):Calories: 144; Total Fat: 2 g; Saturated Fat: 0 g; Cholesterol: 72 mg; Protein: 27 g; Sodium: 59 mg; Potassium: 180 mg; Fiber: 0 g; Carbohydrates: 0 g; Sugar: 0 g

Olive Oil And Lemon Herbed Chicken

Servings: 4

Ingredients:

- 4 (4-ounce) boneless, skinless chicken thighs
- 4 teaspoons olive oil
- 1/8 teaspoon dried marjoram or oregano
- 1/4 teaspoon dried parsley
- 1/8 teaspoon dried rosemary
- 1/8 teaspoon dried thyme or lemon thyme
- 1/4 teaspoon garlic powder
- 2 tablespoons dry white wine
- 1/2 teaspoon cornstarch
- 2 tablespoons fresh lemon juice
- 4 teaspoons margarine

Directions:

1. Add the chicken thighs and olive oil to a heavy-duty, sealable plastic bag. Close the bag and turn it to coat each chicken piece completely.

2. In a small bowl, mix together the marjoram or oregano, parsley, rosemary, thyme, and garlic powder.

3. Heat a nonstick skillet or grill pan over medium-high heat. Remove chicken from marinade; reserve marinade. Dip the top of the chicken in the herb seasoning mixture. Add marinade from the baggie to the skillet. Place the chicken in the skillet, herb-coated-side down.

4. Fry the chicken for 2–3 minutes on each side or until the juices run clear and temperature registers 160°F. Transfer the cooked chicken to a serving platter and keep warm.

5. Add the wine to the skillet, stirring and scraping the bottom of the pan (deglazing) to remove any chicken "bits." Add any herbs remaining in the bowl to the pan. Bring the wine to a boil.

6. Stir the cornstarch into the lemon juice, whisking to remove any lumps. Add the lemon-juice mixture to the wine and bring to a boil. Reduce heat, stirring constantly, simmering the mixture until it thickens.

7. Remove the pan from the heat and whisk in the margarine. Pour over the chicken and serve immediately.

Nutrition Info: (Per Serving):Calories: 101; Total Fat: 6 g; Saturated Fat: 1 g; Cholesterol: 32 mg; Protein: 8 g; Sodium: 34 mg; Potassium: 104 mg; Fiber: 0 g; Carbohydrates: 1 g; Sugar: 0 g

Guacamole-stuffed Chicken

Servings: 4

Ingredients:

- 4 (6-ounce) boneless, skinless chicken breasts
- 1 cup Roasted Garlic Guacamole
- 1/4 cup flour
- 1/8 teaspoon pepper
- 1 large egg, beaten
- 2 slices French Bread , crumbled
- 2 tablespoons grated Parmesan cheese

Directions:

1. Preheat oven to 375°F. Place chicken breasts on waxed paper and cover with more waxed paper. Using a rolling pin, pound until about 1/3" thick, being careful not to tear the meat. Peel off the top piece of waxed paper.
2. Divide guacamole among the chicken breasts and roll up, tucking in the ends. Secure with toothpicks.
3. On plate, combine flour and pepper. Roll chicken in this mixture and shake off excess.

4.   Place egg in shallow bowl. Dip each piece of chicken into the egg.

5.   On plate, combine bread crumbs and cheese. Dip chicken into this mixture to coat and place in baking dish.

6.   Bake chicken for about 30–35 minutes or until a meat thermometer registers 160°F. Make sure you are not putting the thermometer tip in the guacamole in the center of the chicken. Let rest for 5 minutes, then remove toothpicks and serve.

Nutrition Info: (Per Serving):Calories: 291; Total Fat: 10 g; Saturated Fat: 2 g; Cholesterol: 120 mg; Protein: 31 g; Sodium: 140 mg; Potassium: 597 mg; Fiber: 3 g; Carbohydrates: 16 g; Sugar: 0 g

Chicken Curry

Servings: 4

Ingredients:

- 4 teaspoons olive or canola oil
- 4 (4-ounce) boneless, skinless chicken breast fillets
- 1 large Vidalia onion, chopped
- 2 teaspoons curry powder
- 1/4 teaspoon freshly ground black pepper
- 1/8 cup unbleached all-purpose flour
- 1/8 cup unsweetened, no-salt-added applesauce
- 1 cup skim milk

Directions:

1. Bring a large, deep nonstick sauté pan to temperature over medium heat. Add the oil.
2. Add the chicken to the pan and sauté for 2 minutes on each side. Remove from the pan and keep warm.
3. Add the onion and sauté until transparent, about 5 minutes. Add the curry powder and pepper; mix with the onion. Stir in the flour

and applesauce to create a roux. Increase the heat to medium-high.

4. Gradually whisk in the milk, and bring to a boil.

5. Reduce heat to medium-low to maintain a simmer. Add the chicken back to the pan. Cover and simmer for 5 minutes or until the chicken is cooked through to 160°F and the sauce is thickened.

Nutrition Info: (Per Serving):Calories: 208; Total Fat: 6 g; Saturated Fat: 1 g; Cholesterol: 67 mg; Protein: 28 g; Sodium: 107 mg; Potassium: 433 mg; Fiber: 0 g; Carbohydrates: 7 g; Sugar: 4 g

Chili Sauce

Servings: 48

Ingredients:

- 2 cups (475 ml) no-salt-added tomatoes
- 8 ounces (230 g) no-salt-added tomato sauce
- ½ cup (80 g) onion, chopped
- ½ cup (100 g) sugar
- ½ cup (50 g) celery, chopped
- ½ cup (60 g) green bell pepper, chopped
- 1 teaspoon lemon juice
- 1 teaspoon brown sugar
- 1 teaspoon molasses
- ¼ teaspoon hot pepper sauce
- ⅛ teaspoon cloves
- ⅛ teaspoon ground cinnamon
- ⅛ teaspoon black pepper
- ⅛ teaspoon dried basil
- ⅛ teaspoon dried tarragon
- ½ cup (120 ml) cider vi negar

Directions:

1. Combine all ingredients In a large saucepan. Bring to a boil, reduce heat, and simmer uncovered for 1 ½ hours or until the mixture is reduced to half its original volume.

Nutrition Info: (Per Serving): 20 g water; 15 calories (2% from fat, 5% from protein, 94% from carb); 0 g protein; 0 g total fat; 0 g saturated fat; 0 g monounsaturated fat; 0 g polyunsaturated fat; 4 g carb; 0 g fiber; 3 g sugar; 6 mg calcium; 0 mg iron; 3 mg sodium; 56 mg potassium; 39 IU vitamin A; 3 mg vitamin C; 0 mg cholesterol

Fresh Vegetable Pasta Sauce

Servings: 4

Ingredients:

- 2 teaspoons (10 ml) olive oil
- 2 teaspoons (10 ml) lemon juice
- 2 cloves garlic, minced
- 1 teaspoon Italian seasoning
- ¼ teaspoon black pepper
- 2 cups (360 g) tomatoes, chopped
- ½ cup (60 g) green bell pepper, chopped
- 1 cup zucchini, chopped
- ½ cup (80 g) onion, chopped
- ¼ cup (10 g) basil, fresh
- 2 teaspoons (2.6 g) parsley, fresh
- ¼ cup (60 ml) white wine

Directions:

1. In a large skillet, heat olive oil. Add lemon juice, garlic, Italian seasoning, and pepper. Cook until garlic starts to brown. Add vegetables, basil, and parsley and cook until softened. Remove from heat. Stir in wine. Toss with pasta.

Nutrition Info: (Per Serving): 149 g water; 111 calories (58% from fat, 7% from protein, 35% from carb); 2 g protein; 7 g total fat; 1 g saturated fat; 5 g monounsaturated fat; 1 g polyunsaturated fat; 10 g carb; 3 g fiber; 4 g sugar; 81 mg calcium; 2 mg iron; 11 mg sodium; 426 mg potassium; 1126 IU vitamin A; 32 mg vitamin C; 0 mg cholesterol

Sweet Pickled Chipotle Relish (chipotles En Escabèche)

Servings: 3 Cups

Ingredients:

- 4 ounces (about 50) dried chipotle peppers
- Boiling water
- 1 cup cider vinegar
- 1/2 cup packed brown sugar
- 1/2 teaspoon dried thyme
- 1/2 teaspoon dried marjoram
- 3 bay leaves
- 1 medium-size white onion, finely minced
- 1 head garlic, cloves peeled and minced
- 2 teaspoons salt
- 11/4 cups water
- Optional: 1 teaspoon each of celery seeds and mustard seeds

Directions:

1. Put the chipotle peppers in a bowl or jar and pour enough boiling water over them to cover them completely. Keep the peppers submerged and let stand for 10 minutes. Drain

off all the water. If the peppers aren't soft, cover with more boiling water and let stand for an additional 10 minutes. Drain.

2. Remove the stems and discard. Add the peppers to the bowl of a food processor; process until chunky. Drain off most of the liquid, then transfer the peppers to a glass jar that is large enough to comfortably hold all the ingredients and has a noncorrosive lid.

3. In a noncorrosive saucepan, combine all the remaining ingredients. Bring to a gentle simmer and stir until the sugar is completely dissolved, about 5 minutes. Pour the hot liquid over the peppers and stir to mix. The peppers should be completely submerged; if there's not quite enough liquid to cover them, add equal parts cider vinegar and water.

4. Cover and refrigerate for a day or more before serving. This recipe keeps for several weeks in the refrigerator.

Nutrition Info: (Per Serving):Calories: 10; Total Fat: 0 g; Saturated Fat: 0 g; Cholesterol: 0 mg; Protein: 0 g; Sodium: 94 mg; Potassium: 15 mg; Fiber: 0 g; Carbohydrates: 2 g; Sugar: 2 g

Chipotle-poblano Sauce

Servings: 1/2 Cup, 2 Tablespoons

Ingredients:

- 6 chipotle peppers
- 1 poblano pepper
- 1/2 cup boiling water
- 1/2 teaspoon cumin seed
- 1/2 teaspoon dried Mexican oregano
- 1 tablespoon dried minced onion
- 1 teaspoon onion powder
- 2 teaspoons roasted garlic powder
- 1 tablespoon olive oil
- Pinch salt

Directions:

1. Remove the stems and seeds from the peppers, and slit the peppers lengthwise. Roast in a heavy skillet over medium-high heat, turning them occasionally; heat until puffed and just beginning to get brown, about 10 seconds each. (Do not burn the peppers or the resulting sauce will be bitter.) As they're done, put the peppers in a bowl.

2. Pour the boiling water over the peppers; let soak for 15 minutes.

3. Dry-roast the cumin and oregano in the skillet until fragrant, being careful that the oregano doesn't burn.

4. Add the remaining ingredients to the bowl of a food processor or blender container. Process until mixed but still chunky. Leftovers can be stored for several days in the refrigerator.

Nutrition Info: (Per Serving):Calories: 20; Total Fat: 1 g; Saturated Fat: 0 g; Cholesterol: 0 mg; Protein: 0 g; Sodium: 15 mg; Potassium: 44 mg; Fiber: 0 g; Carbohydrates: 1 g; Sugar: 0 g

Honey Mustard Sauce

Servings: 4

Ingredients:

- ¼ cup (85 g) honey
- 2 teaspoons (10 ml) cider vinegar
- 2 teaspoons (10 g) mustard
- ½ teaspoon onion powder
- ¼ teaspoon garlic powder

Directions:

1. Mix ingredients together. Brush over meat when grilling or roasting.

Nutrition Info: (Per Serving): 17 g water; 72 calories (3% from fat, 2% from protein, 95% from carb); 0 g protein; 0 g total fat; 0 g saturated fat; 0 g monounsaturated fat; 0 g polyunsaturated fat; 19 g carb; 0 g fiber; 18 g sugar; 9 mg calcium; 0 mg iron; 4 mg sodium; 35 mg potassium; 10 IU vitamin A; 0 mg vitamin C; 0 mg cholesterol

Fajita Marinade

Servings: 8

Ingredients:

- ¼ cup (60 ml) olive oil
- ¼ cup (60 ml) red wine vinegar
- 2 teaspoons (10 ml) Worcestershire sauce
- 2 teaspoons (10 ml) lemon juice
- 2 teaspoons (10 ml) lime juice
- ½ teaspoon black pepper
- 1 teaspoon cilantro
- 1 teaspoon cumin
- 1 teaspoon garlic powder
- 1 teaspoon dried oregano

Directions:

1. Mix ingredients together and use to marinate beef or chicken for at least 6 hours or overnight.

Nutrition Info: (Per Serving): 15 g water; 70 calories (84% from fat, 2% from protein, 14% from carb); 0 g protein; 7 g total fat; 1 g saturated fat; 5 g monounsaturated fat; 1 g polyunsaturated fat; 3 g carb; 0 g fiber; 1 g sugar; 11 mg calcium; 1 mg iron;

17 mg sodium; 69 mg potassium; 47 IU vitamin A; 10 mg vitamin C; 0 mg cholesterol

Toasted Ground Almonds

Servings: 24

Ingredients:

- 1/2 cup ground raw almonds

Directions:

1. Add the raw almonds to a nonstick skillet over low heat. Toast until golden, shaking the pan or stirring the mixture frequently so that the nuts toast evenly. When the nuts reach a light brown color, remove from the heat and pour into a bowl.

2. Allow to cool completely, then store in an airtight container kept in a cool, dry place.

Nutrition Info: (Per Serving):Calories: 16; Total Fat: 1 g; Saturated Fat: 0 g; Cholesterol: 0 mg; Protein: 0 g; Sodium: 0 mg; Potassium: 20 mg; Fiber: 0 g; Carbohydrates: 0 g; Sugar: 0 g

Guacamole

Servings: 6

Ingredients:

- 1 avocado, peeled and mashed
- 2 teaspoons (6 g) onion, chopped
- 1 teaspoon lime juice
- 1 teaspoon chopped chiles
- ¾ cup (135 g) tomato, peeled and chopped
- ¼ teaspoon garlic powder
- ¼ teaspoon white pepper
- ¼ teaspoon cumin
- ¼ teaspoon cilantro

Directions:

1. Combine all ingredients. Cover and refrigerate for 1 hour to allow flavor to develop.

Nutrition Info: (Per Serving): 44 g water; 55 calories (68% from fat, 6% from protein, 27% from carb); 1 g protein; 5 g total fat; 1 g saturated fat; 3 g monounsaturated fat; 1 g polyunsaturated fat; 4 g carb; 2 g fiber; 1 g sugar; 8 mg calcium; 0 mg iron; 4

mg sodium; 204 mg potassium; 220 IU vitamin A; 9 mg vitamin C; 0 mg cholesterol

Roasted Apple And Onion Relish

Servings: 8

Ingredients:

- 1 small sweet onion, minced
- 1 tart cooking apple, peeled, cored, and chopped
- 1 cup unsweetened, no-salt-added applesauce
- 1 tablespoon apple cider vinegar
- 1 teaspoon frozen apple juice concentrate
- 1 tablespoon lemon juice
- 1/8 teaspoon dried thyme
- 1/8 teaspoon freshly ground black pepper
- Pinch grated orange zest

Directions:

1. Preheat oven to 400°F. Spray a cookie sheet with sides with olive oil spray.
2. Mix together the minced onion and chopped apple; add to the prepared cookie sheet and spread out in a single layer. Lightly spray with olive oil spray. Bake for 10 minutes. Stir the mixture. Bake for 5–10 minutes, until tender and lightly browned.

3. Bring a small nonstick saucepan to temperature over low heat. Add the roasted apple-onion mixture and all of the remaining ingredients; simmer for 15–20 minutes, stirring frequently, until the mixture is reduced by half and light to medium brown in color. Note: Increase the stirring frequency halfway through and until the end of the cooking time, as the relish can easily burn once it's reduced.

4. Cool mixture for 30 minutes, then cover and store in refrigerator.

Nutrition Info: (Per Serving):Calories: 35; Total Fat: 0 g; Saturated Fat: 0 g; Cholesterol: 0 mg; Protein: 0 g; Sodium: 4 mg; Potassium: 92 mg; Fiber: 0 g; Carbohydrates: 9 g; Sugar: 6 g

Sweet And Sour Sauce

Servings: 6

Ingredients:

- ⅓ cup (80 ml) white vinegar
- ½ cup (115 g) brown sugar
- 4 teaspoons (21 g) no-salt-added tomato paste
- ¾ cup (175 ml) water, divided
- 2 teaspoons (3 g) cornstarch

Directions:

1. Mix together the vinegar, sugar, tomato paste, and 1/2 cup (120 ml) of the water. Bring to a boil in a small saucepan. Stir together the cornstarch and remaining water. Add to the other ingredients and continue cooking and stirring until thickened.

Nutrition Info: (Per Serving): 51 g water; 90 calories (0% from fat, 2% from protein, 97% from carb); 0 g protein; 0 g total fat; 0 g saturated fat; 0 g monounsaturated fat; 0 g polyunsaturated fat; 23 g carb; 1 g fiber; 20 g sugar; 21 mg calcium; 1 mg iron; 19 mg sodium; 188 mg potassium; 166 IU vitamin A; 2 mg vitamin C; 0 mg

Tofu-mayo Sandwich Spread

Servings: 1/2 Cup

Ingredients:

- 2 ounces firm silken tofu
- 1/4 cup mayonnaise

Directions:

1. In a small bowl, combine the silken tofu with the mayonnaise. Use as you would mayonnaise. Store in the refrigerator in a covered container until the expiration date on the tofu.

Nutrition Info: (Per Serving):Calories: 53; Total Fat: 5 g; Saturated Fat: 0 g; Cholesterol: 2 mg; Protein: 0 g; Sodium: 39 mg; Potassium: 9 mg; Fiber: 0 g; Carbohydrates: 0 g; Sugar: 0 g

Sun-dried Tomato Vinaigrette

Servings: 8

Ingredients:

- 3 teaspoons (15 ml) white wine vinegar
- ¼ cup (14 g) sun-dried tomatoes, chopped
- 1 teaspoon Worcestershire sauce
- 1 clove garlic, minced
- ½ teaspoon sugar
- ¼ teaspoon white pepper
- ⅓ cup (80 ml) olive oil

Directions:

1. Shake all ingredients together in a jar with a tight-fitting lid.

Nutrition Info: (Per Serving): 8 g water; 90 calories (91% from fat, 1% from protein, 8% from carb); 0 g protein; 9 g total fat; 1 g saturated fat; 7 g monounsaturated fat; 1 g polyunsaturated fat; 2 g carb; 0 g fiber; 1 g sugar; 3 mg calcium; 0 mg iron; 12 mg sodium; 66 mg potassium; 45 IU vitamin A; 5 mg vitamin C; 0 mg cholesterol

Mincemeat-style Chutney

Servings: 48

Ingredients:

- 1 cup diced sweet onion
- 1 cup peeled and diced Granny Smith apples
- 1 cup peeled and diced bananas
- 1 cup peeled and diced peaches
- 1/4 cup raisins
- 1/4 cup dried cranberries
- 1/4 cup dry white wine
- 1/4 cup apple cider vinegar
- 1 teaspoon brown sugar
- 1/2 teaspoon cinnamon
- 1/2 teaspoon Pumpkin Pie Spice
- 1/8 teaspoon freshly ground black pepper
- 1/8 teaspoon grated lemon zest

Directions:

1. In a large saucepan, combine all the ingredients and cook over low heat for about 1 hour, stirring occasionally. Let cool completely. This recipe can be kept in the

refrigerator for 1 week or in the freezer for 3 months.

Nutrition Info: (Per Serving):Calories: 15; Total Fat: 0 g; Saturated Fat: 0 g; Cholesterol: 0 mg; Protein: 0 g; Sodium: 0 mg; Potassium: 43 mg; Fiber: 0 g; Carbohydrates: 3 g; Sugar: 2 g

Barbecue Sauce

Servings: 10

Ingredients:

- ½ cup (120 g) low sodium ketchup
- ½ cup (120 ml) vinegar
- ½ cup (170 g) honey
- ¼ cup (85 g) molasses
- 1 teaspoon chili powder
- 1 teaspoon onion powder
- ½ teaspoon garlic powder
- 1 teaspoon dry mustard
- ¼ teaspoon cayenne pepper

Directions:

1. Combine all ingredients and mix well. Store in a covered jar in the refrigerator.

Nutrition Info: (Per Serving): 24 g water; 97 calories (2% from fat, 2% from protein, 96% from carb); 1 g protein; 0 g total fat; 0 g saturated fat; 0 g monounsaturated fat; 0 g polyunsaturated fat; 25 g carb; 1 g fiber; 22 g sugar; 27 mg calcium; 1 mg iron; 8 mg sodium; 228 mg potassium; 367 IU vitamin A; 3 mg vitamin C; 0 mg cholesterol

Curry Powder

Servings: About 1/4 Cup

Ingredients:

- 1 tablespoon coriander seeds
- 1/2 tablespoon cumin seeds
- 1/2 teaspoon fennel seeds
- 1/4 teaspoon whole cloves or 1/8 teaspoon ground cloves
- 1/4 teaspoon mustard seeds
- 1/2 tablespoon cardamom seeds
- 1/2 tablespoon whole black peppercorns
- 1/2 teaspoon dried red pepper flakes, or crushed red peppers
- 1/2 tablespoon turmeric
- 1/8 teaspoon ground ginger
- 1/8 teaspoon ground cinnamon

Directions:

1. Toast the coriander, cumin, fennel, cloves, mustard seeds, cardamom seeds, peppercorns, and red pepper flakes in a small, dry skillet over medium-low heat. Stir the spices often to prevent them from burning.

Toast for a couple of minutes, or until the spices smell fragrant.

2.   Add the toasted spices to a clean coffee grinder and grind into a fine powder. Add the turmeric, ginger, and cinnamon, and pulse the grinder a few times to combine them with the other spices. Use the spice blend immediately if desired, or, if stored in a sealed glass jar, it can be kept in a cool, dry place for 1 month. To freeze, decant into a hard-sided freezer container and freeze up to 1 year.

Nutrition Info: (Per Serving): (1 tablespoon)Calories: 4; Total Fat: 0 g; Saturated Fat: 0 g; Cholesterol: 0 mg; Protein: 0 g; Sodium: 0 mg; Potassium: 23 mg; Fiber: 0 g; Carbohydrates: 0 g; Sugar: 0 g

Peach Sauce

Servings: 1/2 Cup

Ingredients:

- 2 teaspoons olive oil
- 1 tablespoon chopped shallots
- 1 teaspoon grated fresh ginger
- 1/8 teaspoon grated lemon zest
- 1/2 teaspoon Pumpkin Pie Spice
- Pinch mustard powder
- 1/3 cup dry white wine
- 1 small peach, peeled and diced
- 1 tablespoon frozen orange juice concentrate
- 1 teaspoon Bragg Liquid Aminos
- 1/2 teaspoon cornstarch

Directions:

1. Heat the olive oil in a nonstick saucepan over medium heat; sauté the shallots and ginger until soft.

2. Add the lemon zest, Pumpkin Pie Spice, mustard powder, and wine; simmer until reduced by half.

3. Add the diced peach, orange juice concentrate, and liquid aminos and bring to a simmer, stirring occasionally.

4. In a separate container, mix the cornstarch with 1 tablespoon of the sauce; stir to create a slurry, mixing well to remove any lumps. Add the slurry to the sauce and simmer until the mixture thickens. Transfer the mixture to a blender or food processor container and process until smooth.

Nutrition Info: (Per Serving):Calories: 56; Total Fat: 2 g; Saturated Fat: 0 g; Cholesterol: 0 mg; Protein: 0 g; Sodium: 0 mg; Potassium: 97 mg; Fiber: 0 g; Carbohydrates: 5 g; Sugar: 4 g

Asian Barbecue Sauce

Servings: 16

Ingredients:

- 1 cup (235 ml) Soy Sauce Substitute
- 1 cup (235 ml) water
- 6 teaspoons (30 g) brown sugar
- 2 teaspoons (3.6 g) ground ginger
- 4 teaspoons (20 ml) sesame oil
- 2 teaspoons (10 ml) rice vinegar
- 2 teaspoons (6 g) garlic, minced
- ¼ teaspoon red pepper flakes

Directions:

1. Combine all ingredients and store in a glass jar in the refrigerator for up to 2 weeks.

Nutrition Info: (Per Serving): 16 g water; 31 calories (33% from fat, 0% from protein, 67% from carb); 0 g protein; 1 g total fat; 0 g saturated fat; 0 g monounsaturated fat; 0 g polyunsaturated fat; 5 g carb; 0 g fiber; 5 g sugar; 6 mg calcium; 0 mg iron; 2 mg sodium; 24 mg potassium; 11 IU vitamin A; 0 mgvitamin C; 0 mg cholesterol

Kc Barbecue Sauce

Servings: 24

Ingredients:

- 1 cup (240 g) low sodium ketchup
- 1 cup (245 g) no-salt-added tomato sauce
- ⅔ cup (150 g) brown sugar
- ⅔ cup (157 ml) red wine vinegar
- ¼ cup (85 g) molasses
- 2 teaspoons (10 ml) liquid smoke
- ¼ teaspoon garlic powder
- ¼ teaspoon onion powder
- ¼ teaspoon chili powder
- ½ teaspoon paprika
- ¼ teaspoon celery seed
- ¼ teaspoon ground cinnamon
- ¼ teaspoon cayenne pepper
- ½ teaspoon black pepper, coarsely ground

Directions:

1. In a large saucepan over medium heat, Mix together the ketchup, tomato sauce, brown sugar, wine vinegar, molasses, and liquid smoke. Add garlic powder, onion powder, chili powder, paprika, celery seed, cinnamon,

cayenne pepper, and black pepper. Reduce heat to low and simmer for up to 20 minutes. For thicker sauce, simmer longer, and for thinner, less time is needed.

Nutrition Info: (Per Serving): 23 g water; 49 calories (1% from fat, 2% from protein, 96% from carb); 0 g protein; 0 g total fat; 0 g saturated fat; 0 g monounsaturated fat; 0 g polyunsaturated fat; 13 g carb; 0 g fiber; 11 g sugar; 17 mg calcium; 1 mg iron; 7 mg sodium; 169 mg potassium; 180 IU vitamin A; 3 mg vitamin C; 0 mg cholesterol

Mock Sour Cream

Servings: 6 Tablespoons

Ingredients:

- 2 tablespoons plain nonfat yogurt
- 1/4 cup cottage cheese
- 1/2 teaspoon vinegar

Directions:

1. Put all the ingredients in a blender or food processor; process until smooth.

Nutrition Info: (Per Serving):Calories: 10; Total Fat: 0 g; Saturated Fat: 0 g; Cholesterol: 1 mg; Protein: 1 g; Sodium: 34 mg; Potassium: 20 mg; Fiber: 0 g; Carbohydrates: 0 g; Sugar: 0 g

Jerk Seasoning

Servings: 1/4 Cup

Ingredients:

- 2 teaspoons cayenne pepper
- 1 teaspoon black pepper
- 2 teaspoons onion powder
- 2 teaspoons garlic powder
- 2 teaspoons sugar
- 1 teaspoon smoked paprika
- 1 teaspoon dried thyme leaves
- 1/2 teaspoon ground allspice
- 1/4 teaspoon cardamom
- 1/4 teaspoon nutmeg

Directions:

1. Combine all ingredients in small bowl and mix well. Store in tightly covered jar at room temperature.

Nutrition Info: (Per Serving):Calories: 6; Total Fat: 0 g; Saturated Fat: 0 g; Cholesterol: 0 mg; Protein: 0 g; Sodium: 0 mg; Potassium: 22 mg; Fiber: 0 g; Carbohydrates: 1 g; Sugar: 0 g

Teriyaki Sauce Substitute

Servings: 20

Ingredients:

- 1 cup (235 ml) Soy Sauce Substitute
- 2 teaspoons (10 ml) sesame oil
- 2 teaspoons (10 ml) sake
- ½ cup (100 g) sugar
- 3 cloves garlic, crushed
- 1 teaspoon gingerroot, minced
- Dash black pepper

Directions:

1. Combine all ingredients in a saucepan and heat until sugar is dissolved. Store in the refrigerator.

Nutrition Info: (Per Serving): 1 g water; 35 calories (36% from fat, 0% from protein, 63% from carb); 0 g protein; 1 g total fat; 0 g saturated fat; 1 g monounsaturated fat; 1 g polyunsaturated fat; 5 g carb; 0 g fiber; 5 g sugar; 1 mg calcium; 0 mg iron; 0 mg sodium; 4 mg potassium; 0 IU vitamin A; 0 mg vitamin C; 0 mg cholesterol

Slow Cooker Caramelized Onions

Servings: 6

Ingredients:

- 5 large onions, sliced
- 2 tablespoons olive oil
- 1 teaspoon lemon juice
- 1/8 teaspoon white pepper

Directions:

1. Combine all ingredients in a 4-quart slow cooker.
2. Cover and cook on low for 8–10 hours, stirring occasionally, until the onions are deep golden brown and very soft. If the mixture is liquid, set the lid ajar and cook on low for another hour or two until the liquid evaporates.
3. Cover and refrigerate up to 3 days, or freeze in 1/4-cup portions for up to 6 months.

Nutrition Info: (Per Serving):Calories: 86; Total Fat: 4 g; Saturated Fat: 0 g; Cholesterol: 0 mg; Protein: 1 g; Sodium: 3 mg; Potassium: 178 mg; Fiber: 1 g; Carbohydrates: 10 g; Sugar: 5 g

Mustard

Servings: 36

Ingredients:

- ¼ cup (36 g) dry mustard
- ¼ cup (60 ml) white wine vinegar
- ¼ cup (60 ml) white wine
- 1 teaspoon sugar
- 1 egg yolk

Directions:

1. Blend together all the ingredients except the egg yolk and let stand for 2 hours. Beat the egg yolk into the mixture. Cook, stirring constantly, until slightly thickened, about 5 minutes. Store covered in the refrigerator.

Nutrition Info: (Per Serving): Each with: 7 g water; 5 calories (29% from fat, 36% from protein, 35% from carb); 0 g protein; 0 g total fat; 0 g saturated fat; 0 g monounsaturated fat; 0 g polyunsaturated fat; 0 g carb; 0 g fiber; 0 g sugar; 3 mg calcium; 0 mg iron; 5 mg sodium; 14 mg potassium; 12 IU vitamin A; 0 mg vitamin C; 0 mg cholesterol

Duxelles

Servings: 2 Cups

Ingredients:

- 2 tablespoons unsalted butter
- 1 tablespoon olive oil
- 1 pound cremini mushrooms, chopped
- 1/2 pound portobello mushrooms, chopped
- 1 medium onion, chopped
- 4 cloves garlic, minced
- 1 tablespoon red wine
- 2 tablespoons lemon juice
- 3 tablespoons heavy cream
- 1 teaspoon dried marjoram leaves
- 1/8 teaspoon pepper

Directions:

1. In a medium skillet, heat butter and olive oil over medium heat. Add cremini mushrooms, portobello mushrooms, onion, and garlic. Reduce heat to low.
2. Cook, stirring frequently, until the mushrooms give up their liquid and the liquid evaporates, about 7–8 minutes. Continue

cooking and stirring until the mushrooms are deep brown, about 20–30 minutes longer.

3.   Add wine, lemon juice, cream, marjoram, and pepper, and simmer for 5 minutes longer.

4.   Mixture can be refrigerated up to 1 week, or frozen in 2-tablespoon portions for up to 3 months.

Nutrition Info: (Per Serving): (2 tablespoons)Calories: 43; Total Fat: 3 g; Saturated Fat: 1 g; Cholesterol: 7 mg; Protein: 1 g; Sodium: 4 mg; Potassium: 204 mg; Fiber: 0 g; Carbohydrates: 2 g; Sugar: 0 g

Lightning Source UK Ltd.
Milton Keynes UK
UKHW051522270721
387836UK00006B/84